Contents

1 How to Become a Make-up Artist

Becky has won a make-over in a competition.
She is keen to be a make-up artist herself.
She takes the chance to ask Meera,
the make-up artist, about her job.

Meera: Right Becky, sit in the treatment chair.
Just relax. I'm going to start
by cleansing your skin.
After that I'll give you a mini-facial.
Then we'll choose the look you want
for your new make-up.

Becky: That sounds great.
I'd like to do this sort of work myself.
Do you mind if I ask you about your job?

Meera: Not at all. But you'll have to keep still
while I tidy your eyebrows,
put your lipstick on and so on.

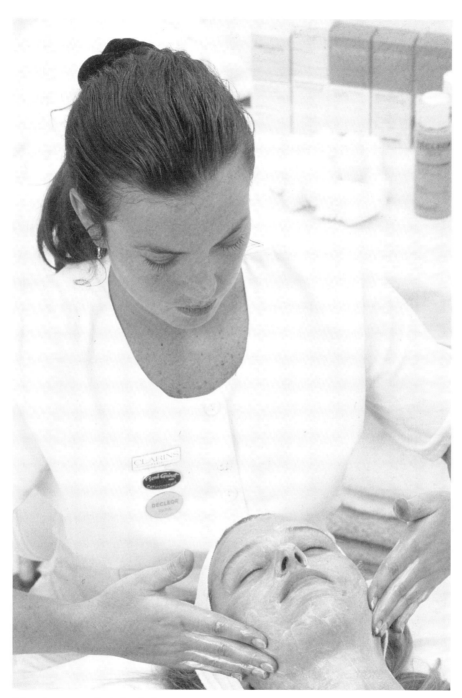

Having a mini-facial.

Becky: How do I go about getting a job like yours?
Would I need to go to college?

Meera: There aren't any courses for make-up artists.
Most people begin by doing a course in
beauty therapy.
There are lots of different jobs to choose
from once you've done that.

Becky: Would I need good exam results to get
on a college course?

Meera: That depends on the college
– and the sort of course it offers.
Check out your local one.
Most college courses last two years.
They lead to an NVQ at Level 2.

It's best to aim for some GCSEs.
English and maths are worth having.
Biology is useful for beauty therapy.

You need to know about the human body.
If you do want to be a make-up artist,
art is always a good choice.
It helps if you have an eye for colour.

Becky: That's lucky. Art is my best subject.
How does it help in beauty therapy?

Meera: When I first meet a client I take note
of the colour of her hair and her eyes.
I also look at her skin tone.

You have fair skin so you'd look best
in cool shades like blue and grey.
The make-up I'll choose for you
must match those tones.

I couldn't wear the same shades myself.
My skin is too dark.
I need warm shades.
At one time it was hard for black
and Asian girls to find the right make-up.
There's quite a good range now.

Becky: What else do you learn at college?

Meera: You learn about different skin types.
How to do facials and apply make-up
– both for day and evening.
How to tint eyelashes and shape eyebrows.
How to remove unwanted hair.
You learn how to care for hands and feet,
– do a manicure and a pedicure.
How to give a massage.
But there are other skills you need as well.

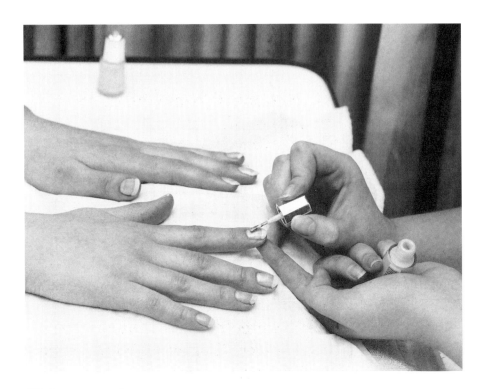

Giving a manicure.

Becky: That's quite a list already!
What other skills do you mean?

Meera: You have to be able to deal with clients
from all walks of life.
Not all of them are nice to you.
You can get some awkward ones.

Becky: Oh dear! How do you cope with them?

Meera: You have to be very tactful.
You must also learn to put shy people
at their ease.
A lot of clients aren't very confident.
Some of them aren't happy with their looks.
That's why they come to us.

They may want to play down a bad point,
– such as a big nose.
They may have a scar they want to hide,
or cover up really bad skin.

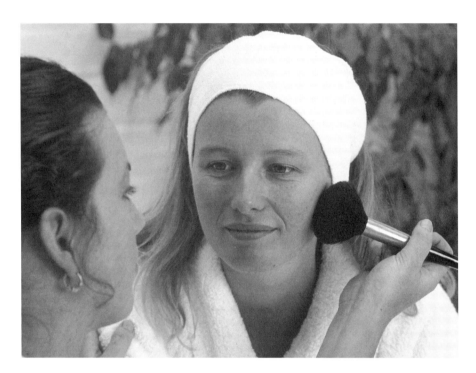

Having a make-over.

On the other hand, some women just want
to look good for a special day …
for a wedding or a party.
Or like you, they come to learn
how to apply make-up.
I show them how to get
the best effects at home.

Becky: Yes, I was hoping to pick up
some tips from you today.

Meera: People need to feel they can trust you,
and you must be gentle.
Some of the treatments hurt a bit.
Like when you pluck eyebrows
or wax someone's legs.

Meera: A lot of clients are older women.
You've got to make them look good
but with styles that suit their age.
You don't have to panic
if something goes wrong.
You just need to know how to put it right.

Becky: That seems a lot to remember …
Is there anything else?

Meera:	Well, you're working close to people,
	doing very personal things for them.
	You've got to look smart and stay fresh.
	Your own personal hygiene is
	very important.
	So is your attitude.
Becky:	How do you mean?
Meera:	You've got to be professional at all times.
	Know when a client wants to chat
	– and when she wants to be quiet.
	She may tell you about her private life.
	You mustn't repeat what she's said.
	Don't ever spread gossip about your clients.
Becky:	Oh dear, there seems an awful lot to take in.
Meera:	There is, but you'll learn it all in time.
	Another part of our course was
	business studies.
	You may own your own salon one day,
	or at least manage one.
	You need to know all about costing and
	working to a budget.
	That's when the maths
	is really needed.

Becky: Is there anything else?

Meera: One very important thing.
How's your health?

Becky: OK I guess. I'm pretty fit.
Why do you ask?

Meera: Because you need stamina in this job.
You're on your feet for hours on end.
There's a lot of standing about.
Giving a massage can be quite tiring.

Meera: There, I've finished your facial.
I haven't any other clients today.
Let's take a break and have a coffee.
Then I'll show you how to apply
your make-up.
We can talk some more later.

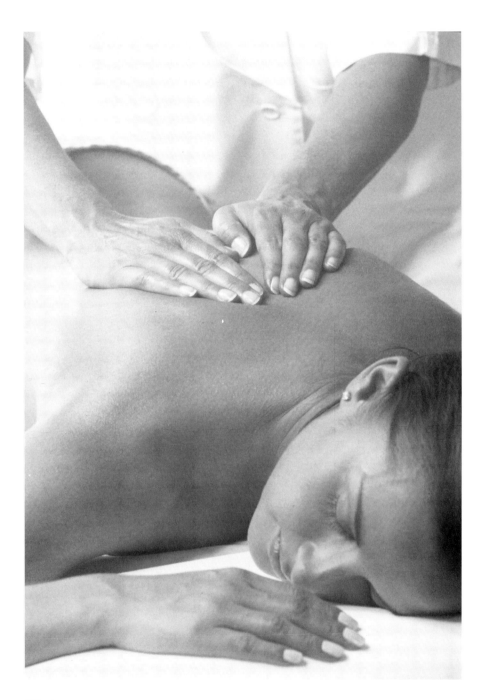

Giving a massage.

Becky: My skin feels great. Really soft and smooth.
I don't spend nearly as much time as that
cleaning my face at home.

Meera: That's a mistake a lot of girls make.
It pays to keep your skin
in good condition.
Massage it with your finger tips,
the way I did.
Get it deep-down clean.
Drink plenty of water.
That helps to keep it clear.

Make sure all the things you put near
your face are really clean too.
Always check your brushes and sponges.
Throw them away if they look grubby.

2 Getting a Job

Meera: Right, shall we make you beautiful?
What kind of make-up do you want?
A look for day time or a bit of glamour
for an evening out?

Becky: I don't really wear much make-up
in the day time.
We can't wear it at school
and I play sport most weekends.
I'd like a really special look,
something for a party or a disco.
I'm going to one tonight.

Meera: OK. Have a look in my make-up tray.
See what you fancy.
These eye shadows are new this season.
The pinky shades would suit you.
What about a darker lipstick?
There's one in plum I quite like.
I'll also put a bit of this glitter
along your cheek bones.

Becky: Some of these colours are lovely.
Do they cost a lot?

Meera: These are quite dear.
They're the sort I use
on models in photo sessions.
But you can buy some good make-up
quite cheaply in the chain stores now.
Or even in the local supermarkets.
You don't need to spend a fortune.

Becky: You said you'd tell me more about
your work.
Did you get a job
as soon as you left college?

Meera: Yes, but it wasn't a very glamorous one.
I worked in a friend's salon.
She was the hairdresser.
I did everything else.
I made the tea, answered the phone.
Washed the clients' hair
and swept the floor.

Now and again I did a manicure.
I worked there for a year before I got
a better job.
The pay was low but it was
good experience.

Becky: What was your next job?

Meera: That was a bit more upmarket.
It was in a salon in the West End.
I did the full range
of beauty treatments there.
It still wasn't all that well paid
but I got some good tips.
I built up my own list of clients
who asked for me by name.

Becky: Do most make-up artists start off
working in a salon?

Meera: A lot of them do.
But as I told you, there are
quite a few jobs open to you
once you've done the basic course.

I kept in touch with some of the girls
who did beauty therapy at college.
They had quite a range of jobs.

Becky: What sort of jobs?

Meera: Sue went to work in a big store.
She became a rep for a cosmetic firm.
Her job was to show women
how to use their products.

It was well paid but she worked hard.
A lot of clients booked in at lunch times
or after work.

There were some good perks with the job.
She got discounts on goods she bought
in the store.

Cheetal wanted to work abroad.
She got a job in a top hotel in Paris.
She had a life of luxury.
Good food and a lovely room
but she was on duty every day.
A lot of rich women expect the staff
to be on hand at all times.

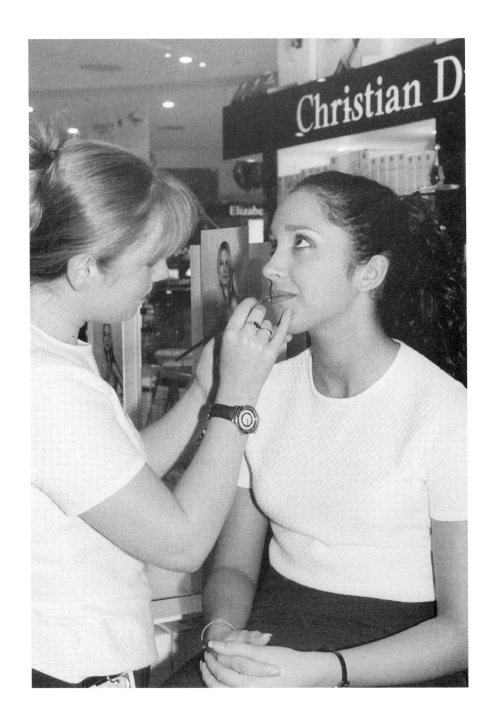

Working in a big London store.

Kim went to work at a health farm.
She had to learn how to do
special treatments.
Steam baths, mud packs and so on.

The health farm was way out in the country
so she didn't get much social life.
But she could use things like the jacuzzi
and the sauna for free.

Then there was Carol.
She went to work on board ship.
On a cruise liner.
She didn't do it for long though.

Becky: Why was that?

Meera: She fell in love with one of the crew
on her very first trip.
They got married soon after.
She's got two children now.
She sells cosmetics door to door.

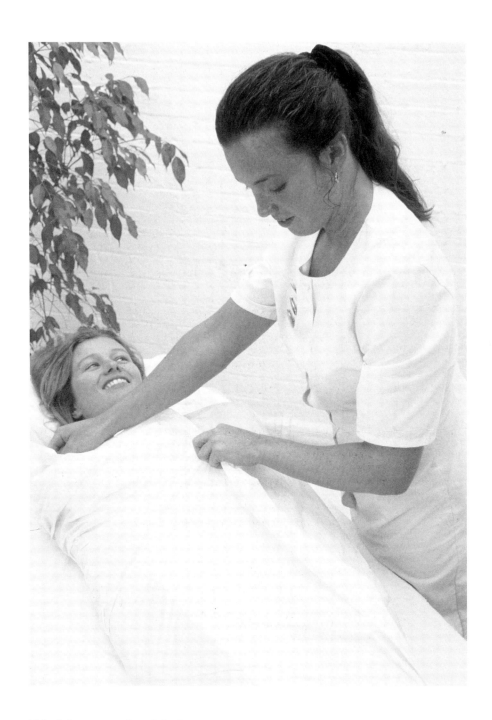

Working on a health farm.

Becky: What about you, Meera?
How did you come to be a make-up artist?

Meera: By chance really.

Meera: My sister saw an advert in a trade paper.
A TV company wanted staff to train
for work in television.
I wrote off and got an interview.

Becky: Are there many schemes like that?

Meera: Not many. I think the BBC runs one
but it's hard to get on it.
Lots of people apply but they only take on
a few each year.

Becky: It must have been exciting,
working in TV.
Did you make up many famous people?

Meera: Not at first. When I started I was
just the assistant.
I had to check all the trays.
Set things up for the make-up artists.
Then I had to order new stock
if we were running low.

I spent a lot of time getting people
ready to face the cameras.
Ordinary people who'd come in to do
interviews on news items.
I had to powder their noses – or bald heads!
So they didn't shine too much on screen.

Then I began to learn the tricks of the trade.
How to do special effects make-up.
Programmes like *Casualty*
rely on their make-up artists.
If we did a hospital scene we had
to make fake scars from wax and
paint cuts and bruises on the actors.

The filming may last a few days.
If they have to shoot the scene again
you make a note of where to put
the scars the next day.
They have to be in the same place.

For drama there was quite a lot to learn.
In a soap the actor's hair and make-up
must always look the same.
Sometimes in a play an actor has to age.

He might start off as a young man
and finish up many years older.
It takes a lot of work in make-up
to make that look real.
You have to make up his hands too.
The body ages as well as the face.

If a drama's set in the past,
you have to be able to do the styles
that were in fashion at the time.
You spend a lot of time on the hair.
Dressing wigs, putting on false beards,
and so on.

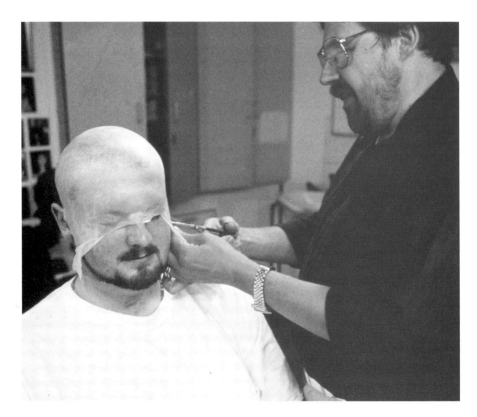

Creating a bald head.

Becky: I was going to ask you about that.
Do you need to learn hairdressing?

Meera: You don't have to cut hair
but you need to be able to style it.

Becky: What other programmes did you work on?

Meera: I once worked on a Sci-Fi series.
That was quite fun.
I got to do some fantasy make-up.
It was set in the future so the actors
had to look very weird.
They were meant to be from another planet.

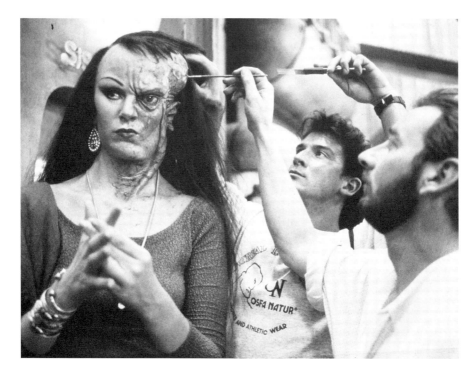

Fantasy make-up from *Total Recall*.

Becky: How long did you work for the
TV company?

Meera: A couple of years.
I enjoyed it but I wanted a change.
When I got the chance to work in films
I went freelance.

Becky: What does that mean?

Meera: It means you're your own boss.
You don't work for one company.
I knew a lot of people.
Had a lot of contacts.
So I got plenty of work.

Being freelance means
I get a variety of jobs.
I might work on a film one week,
a fashion show the next.
I also do make-up for adverts on TV
and magazines.

I enjoy the buzz and I get to travel.
Next month I'm working on a film.
It's on location in Africa.

Becky: That sounds great.

Meera: It's not all fun on location.
You have to be up really early
to get the actors ready for filming.

There's a lot of standing about
waiting to touch up their make-up.
Sometimes the weather's bad.
You have to make them look sun-tanned
even if it's been pouring with rain.

Becky: Is that sort of work well paid?

Meera: It can be. It all depends.
As you become better known
you get bigger fees.
There's a big demand for people
to do special effect make-up.
Think of Freddy Kruger in
Nightmare on Elm Street.
All the characters in the *Batman* films.

Now, what do you think?
Does that look OK?
Are you happy with your new look?

Becky: It's perfect. Thanks a lot, Meera.
And thanks for taking the time
to answer all my questions.

Meera: I'm glad to be of help.
I've enjoyed our chat, Becky.
I hope you make it one day.
I'll look out for your name on the credits
at the end of TV shows.

Useful Addresses

British Association of Beauty Therapy and
Cosmetology Ltd.
Parabola House
Parabola Road
Cheltenham
GL50 3AH

British Industry Authority (BIA)
3 Chequer Road
Doncaster
South Yorkshire
DN1 2AA
(For information on NVQs)

Film and Television Freelance Training (FT2)
4th Floor
Warwick House
9 Warwick Street
London
W1R SRA